Date: 9/1/20

J 610.69 HAN
Hansen, Grace,
Heroes of COVID-19 /

Heroes of COVID-19

by Grace Hansen

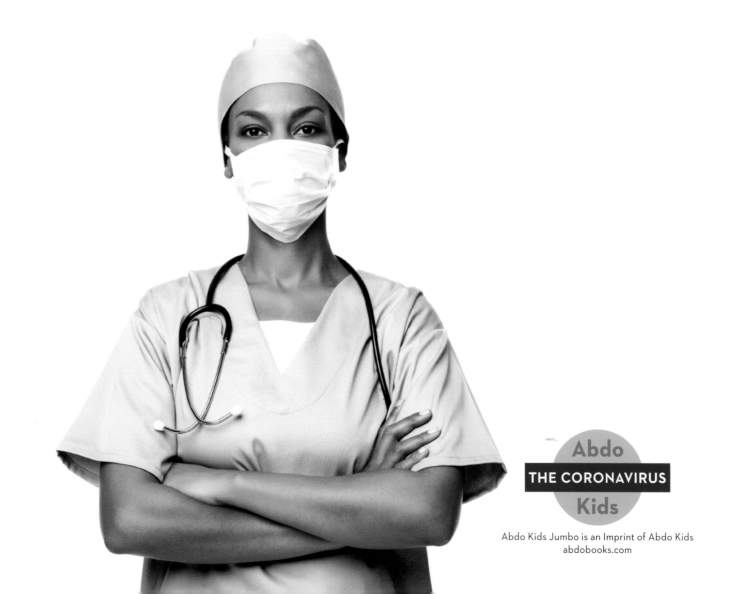

Abdo
THE CORONAVIRUS
Kids

Abdo Kids Jumbo is an Imprint of Abdo Kids
abdobooks.com

abdobooks.com

Published by Abdo Kids, a division of ABDO, P.O. Box 398166, Minneapolis, Minnesota 55439.
Copyright © 2021 by Abdo Consulting Group, Inc. International copyrights reserved in all countries.
No part of this book may be reproduced in any form without written permission from the publisher.
Abdo Kids Jumbo™ is a trademark and logo of Abdo Kids.

Printed in the United States of America, North Mankato, Minnesota.

052020

092020

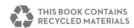
THIS BOOK CONTAINS
RECYCLED MATERIALS

Photo Credits: AP Images, Getty Images, iStock, Shutterstock, ©Shutterstock PREMIER p.Cover

Production Contributors: Teddy Borth, Jennie Forsberg, Grace Hansen
Design Contributors: Dorothy Toth, Pakou Moua

Library of Congress Control Number: 2020936703
Publisher's Cataloging-in-Publication Data

Names: Hansen, Grace, author.

Title: Heroes of COVID-19 / by Grace Hansen

Description: Minneapolis, Minnesota : Abdo Kids, 2021 | Series: The Coronavirus | Includes online
    resources and index.

Identifiers: ISBN 9781098205522 (lib. bdg.) | ISBN 9781098205669 (ebook) | ISBN 9781098205737
    (Read-to-Me ebook)

Subjects: LCSH: Medical personnel--Juvenile literature. | Food service employees--Juvenile literature. |
    School employees--Juvenile literature. | Volunteers--Juvenile literature. | Heroes--Juvenile literature. |
    Epidemics--Juvenile literature.

Classification: DDC 610.69--dc23

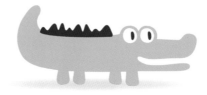

Table of Contents

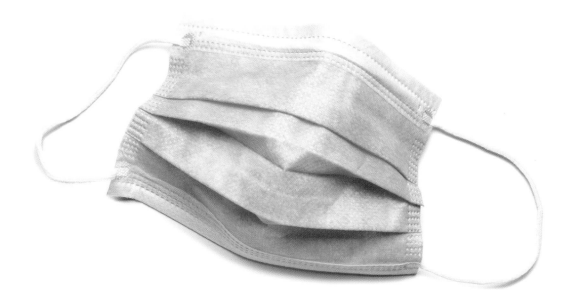

COVID-19

COVID-19 is short for

Coronavirus Disease 2019.

The illness spreads very easily

from person to person. To

slow the spread, people had

to stay away from each other.

4

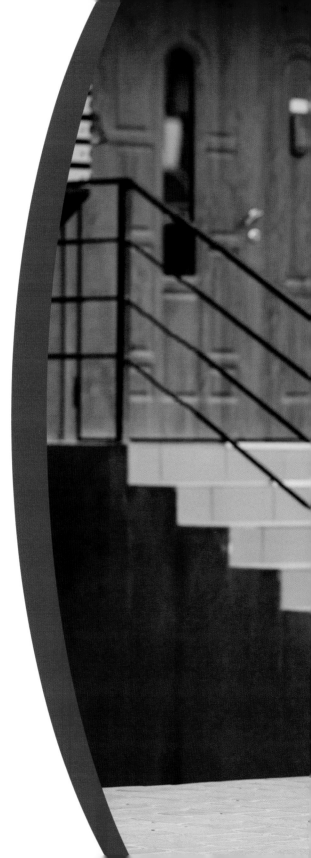

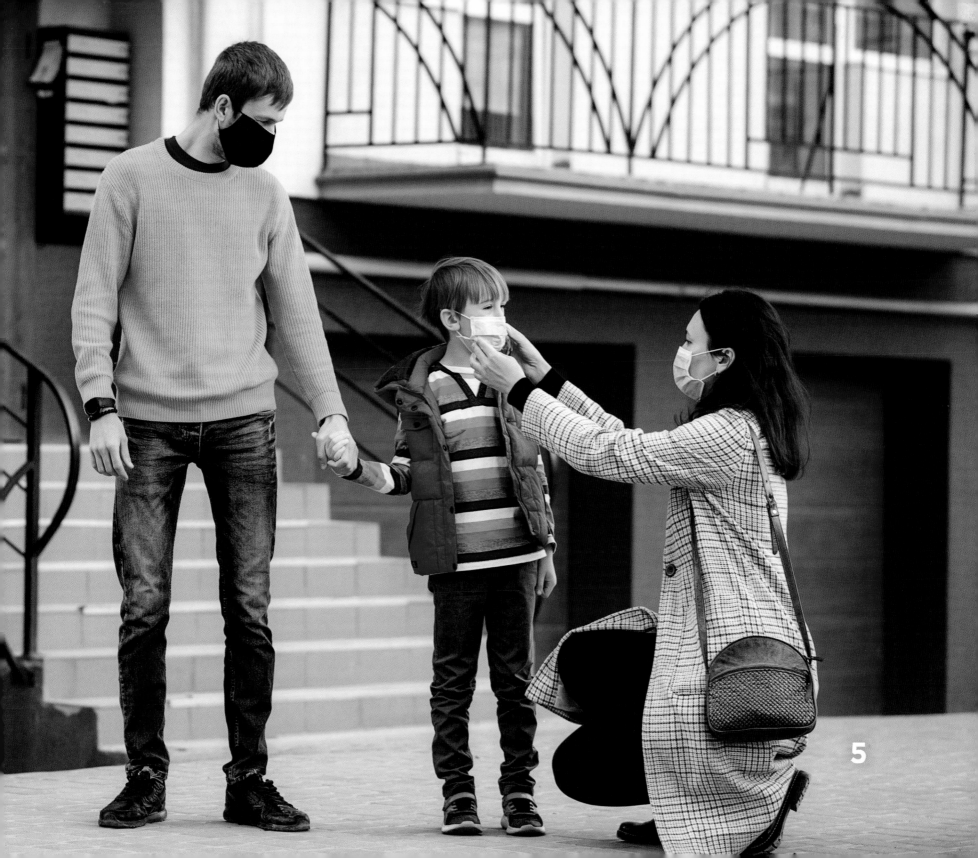

Many businesses had to shut down. However, lots of people still went to work each day. Without **essential** workers, things would have been much worse.

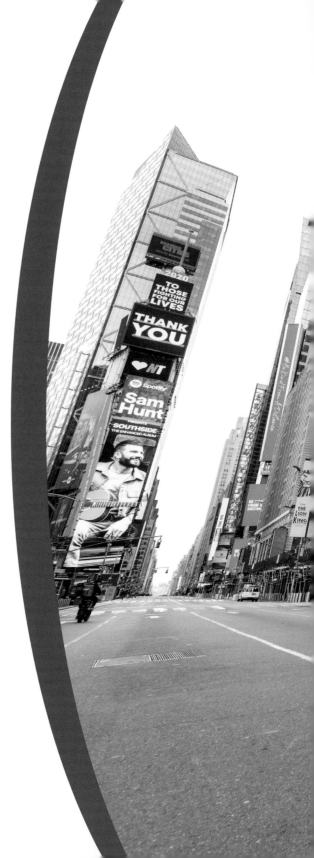

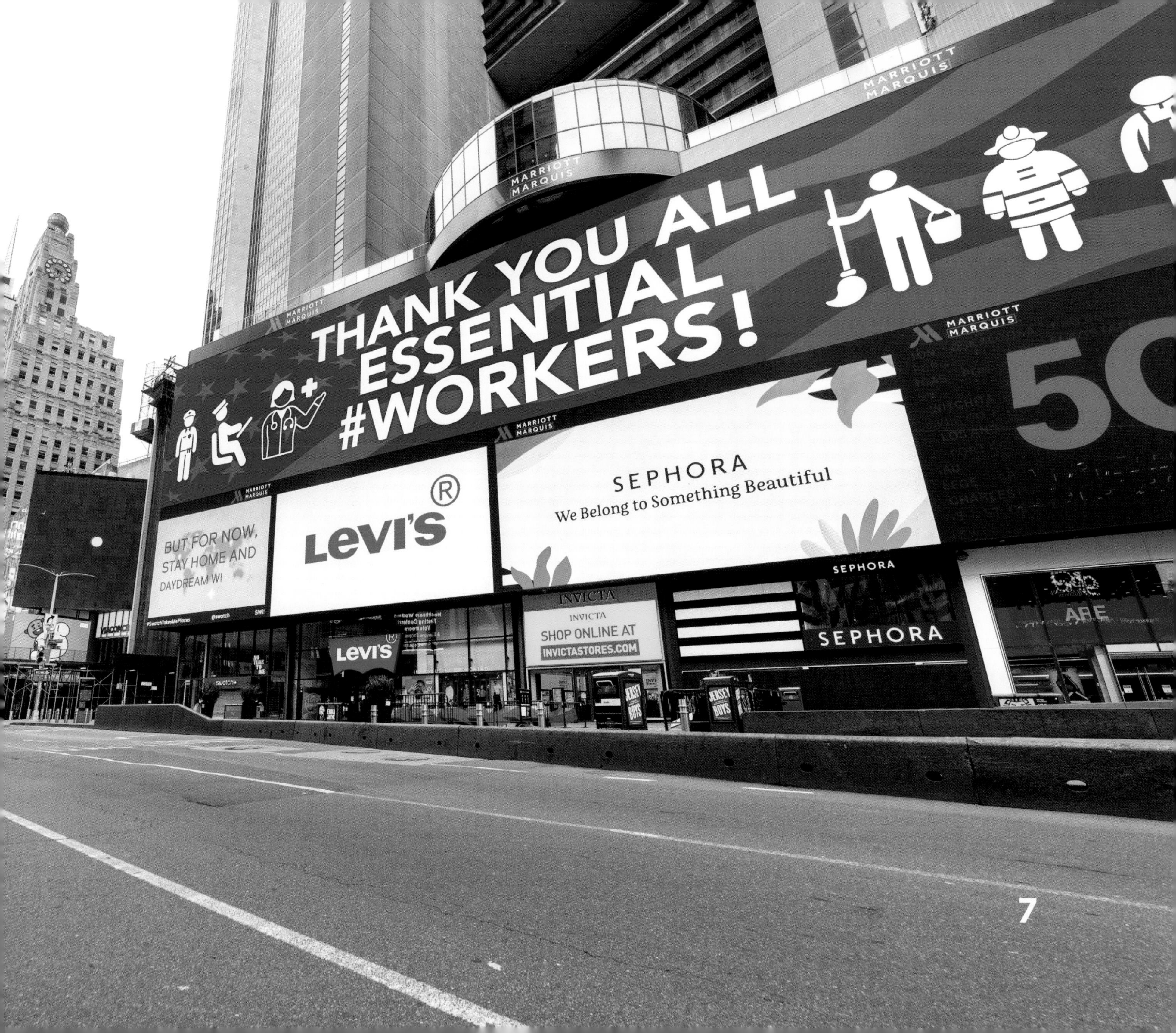
MARRIOTT MARQUIS
THANK YOU ALL
ESSENTIAL
#WORKERS!
BUT FOR NOW,
STAY HOME AND
DAYDREAM WI
Levi's
SEPHORA
We Belong to Something Beautiful
INVICTA
SHOP ONLINE AT
INVICTASTORES.COM
SEPHORA

Essential Workers

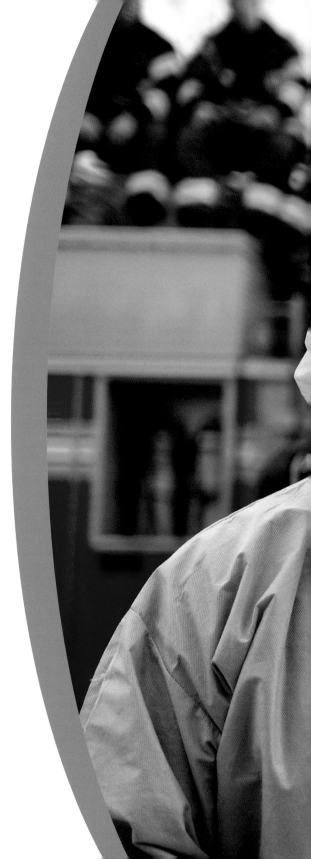

Health care workers risked their own health to save others. **Paramedics** brought sick patients safely to hospitals. Doctors and nurses cared for the ill.

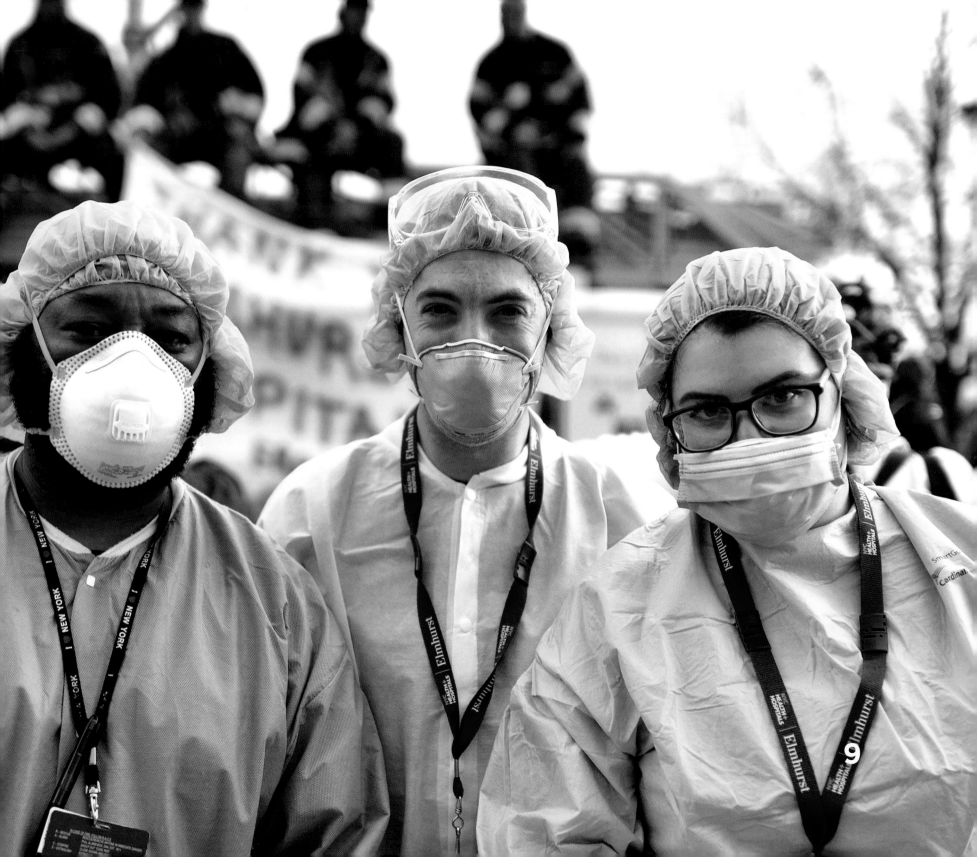

Farmers and farmworkers still grew and gathered food. Grocery store workers stocked shelves.

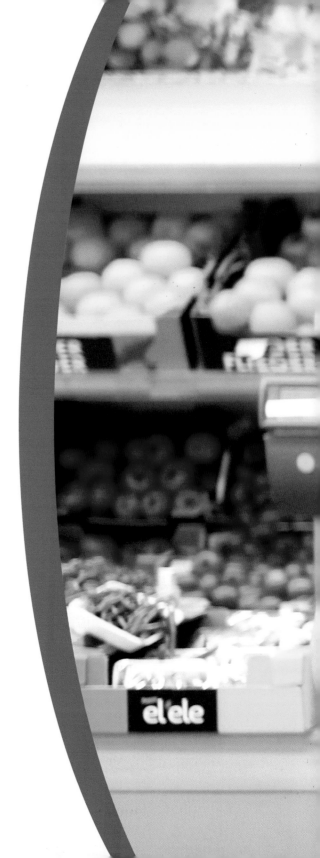

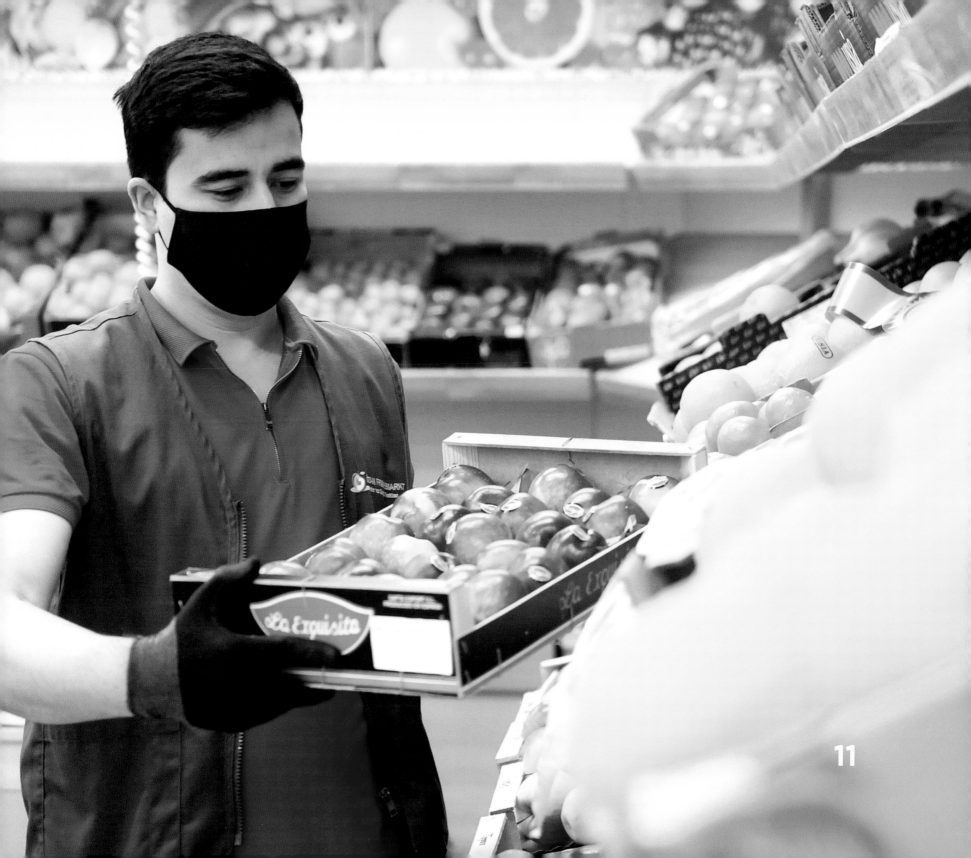

Public transit workers got people where they needed to go. Truck drivers brought goods to stores. Delivery people drove items to people's homes.

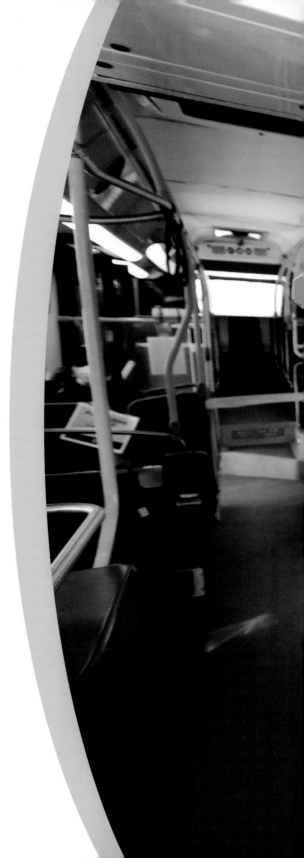

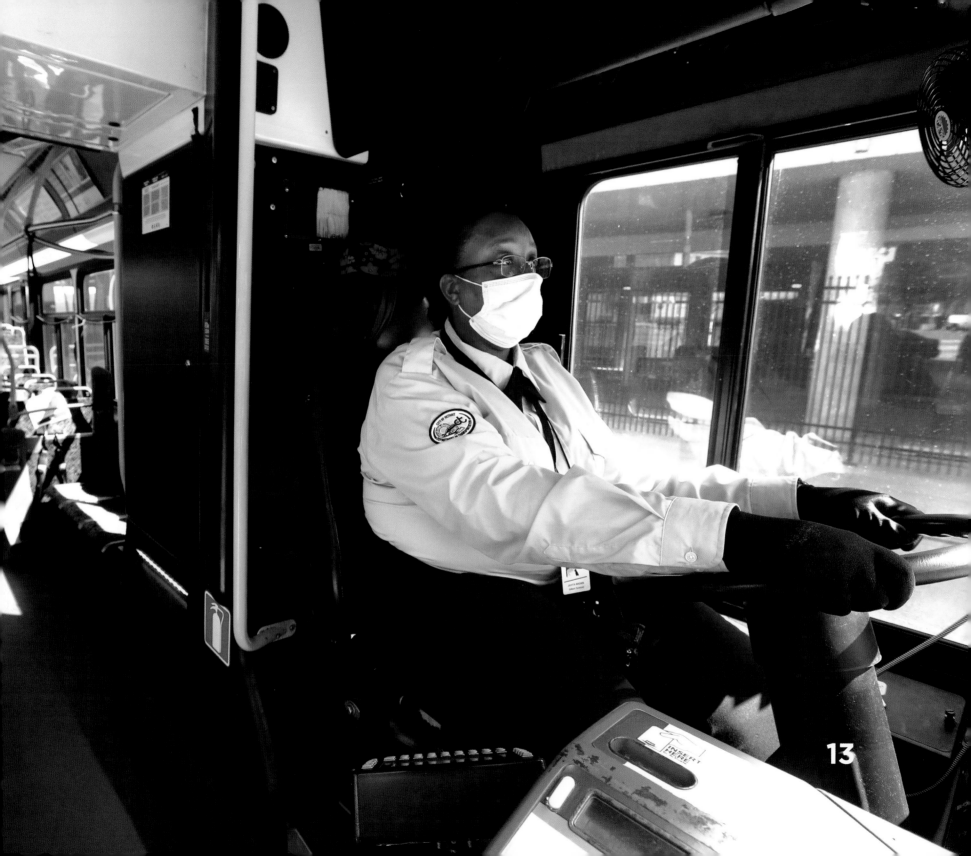

13

Manufacturer workers helped make more paper products. They made cleaning supplies and other needed items. Warehouse workers packed and shipped the items.

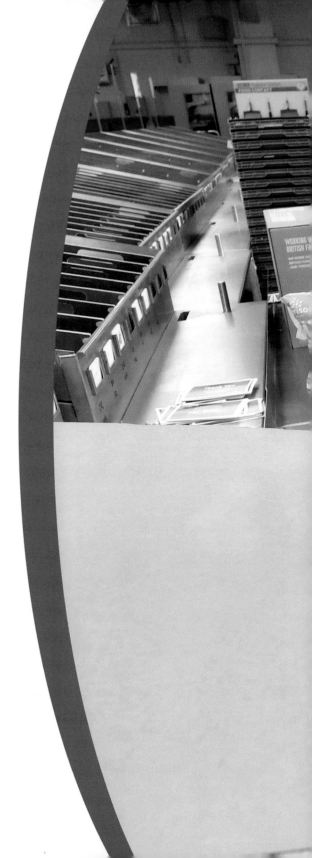

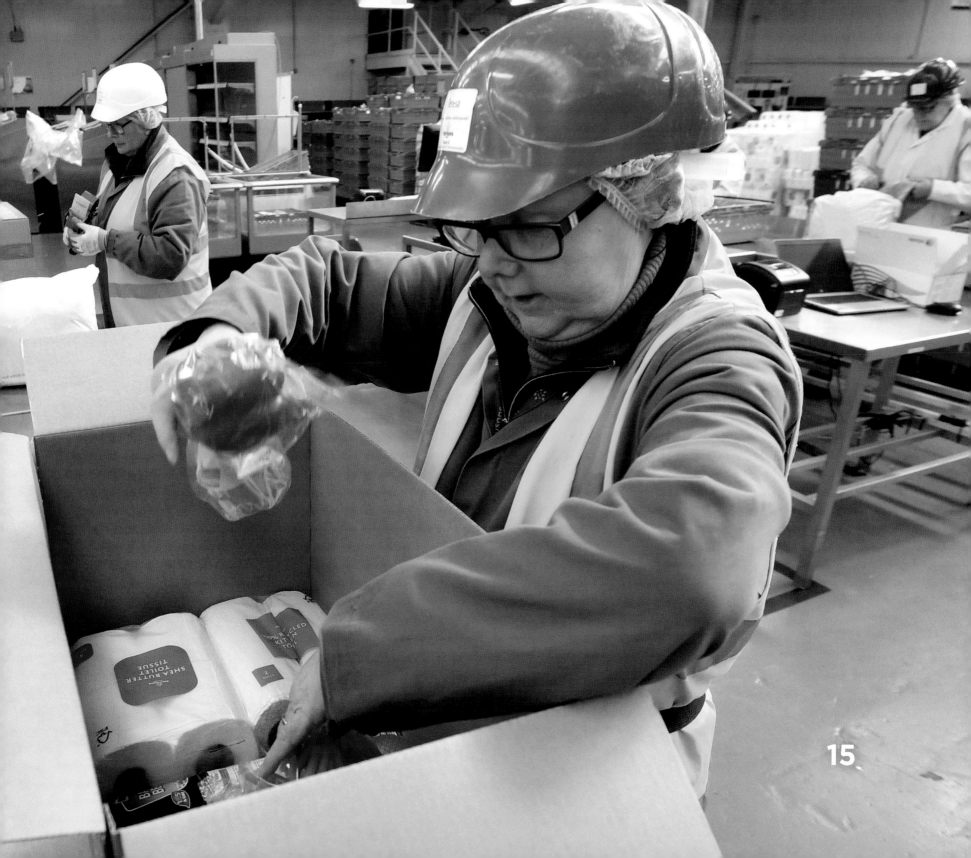

Schools and educators had to get creative. Teachers found new ways for students to learn from home.

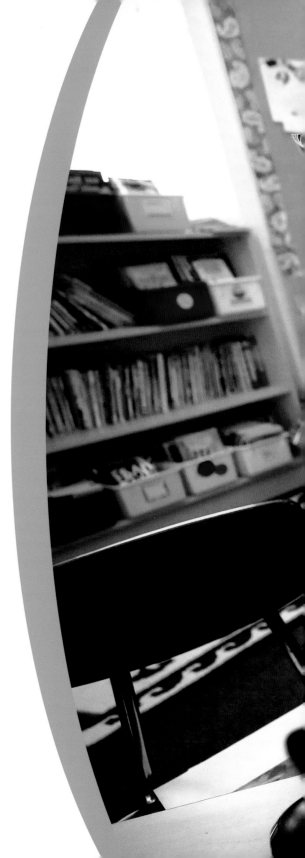

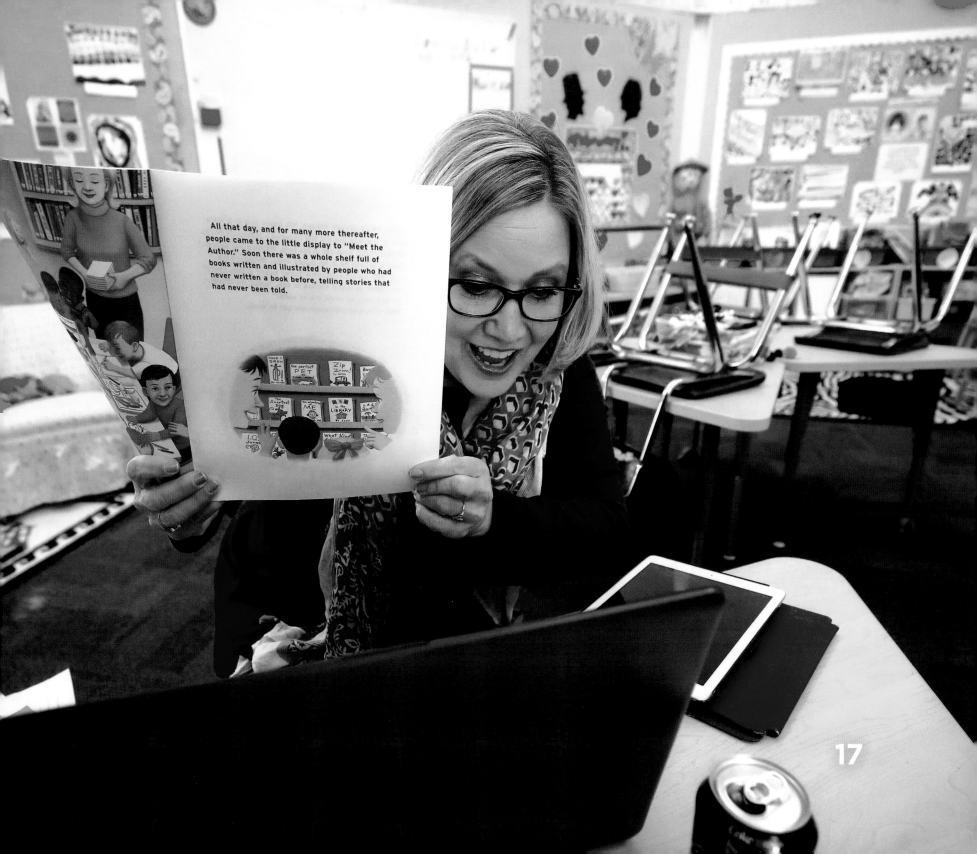

All that day, and for many more thereafter, people came to the little display to "Meet the Author." Soon there was a whole shelf full of books written and illustrated by people who had never written a book before, telling stories that had never been told.

Governors and mayors helped their states and towns. They educated people about COVID-19. They guided their citizens to help stop the spread.

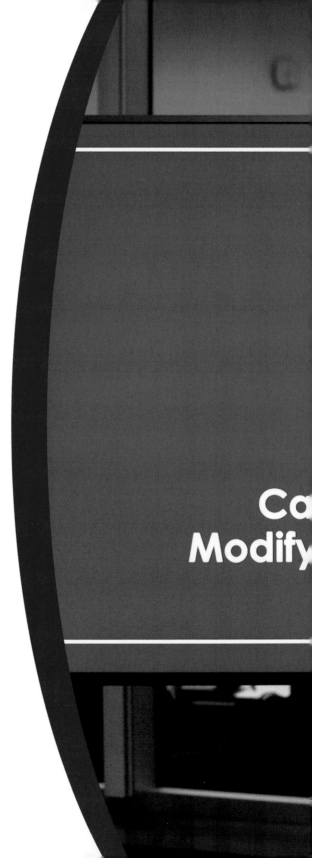

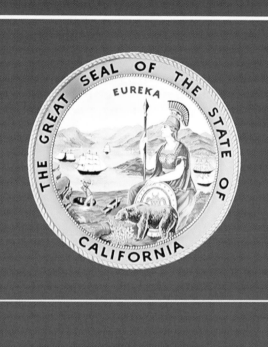

ornia's Roadmap to
he Stay-at-Home Order

19

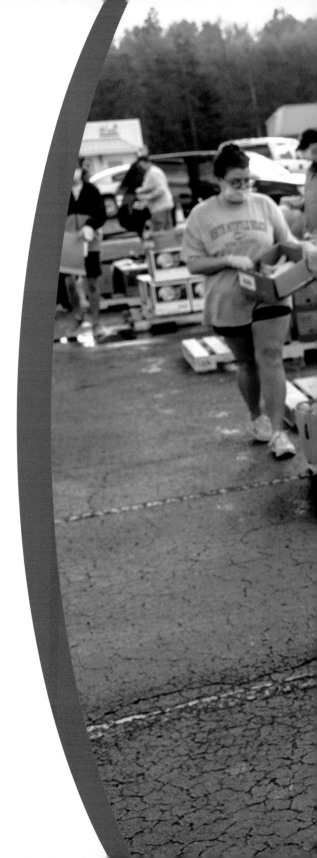

Volunteers handed out food to those in need. Things were not easy during this time. But many people still stepped up to help!

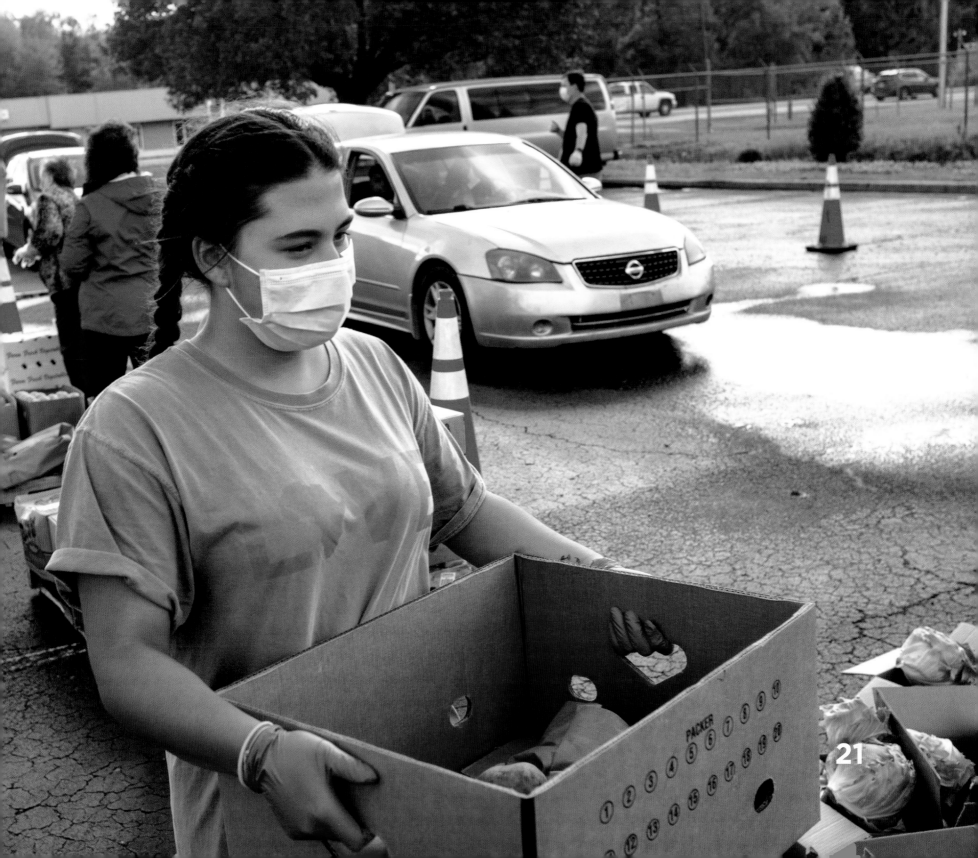

More Information About COVID-19

- COVID-19 is short for <u>Co</u>rona<u>v</u>irus <u>D</u>isease 20<u>19</u>.

- COVID-19 is an illness caused by a coronavirus strain called SARS-CoV-2. People do not have any **immunity** to the virus.

- SARS-CoV-2 is short for Severe Acute Respiratory Syndrome Coronavirus 2.

- Common symptoms of COVID-19 include cough, fever, and shortness of breath.

Glossary

coronavirus – any of a group of viruses that cause disease. In humans, most coronaviruses cause illnesses like the common cold. Others cause more serious illnesses.

essential – extremely important and necessary.

immunity – the ability to resist a certain virus by the action of certain antibodies.

manufacturer – a company that makes things in large quantities.

paramedic – one who is trained to work as a doctor's assistant or as a provider of emergency medical care.

volunteer – a person who offers to work or help without pay.

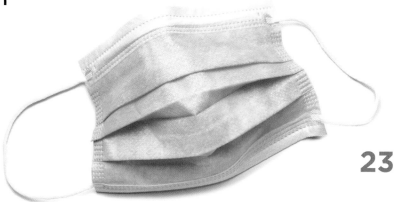

Index

 Abdo Kids ONLINE FREE! ONLINE MULTIMEDIA RESOURCES

Visit **abdokids.com** to access crafts, games, videos, and more!

Use Abdo Kids code **THK5515** or scan this QR code!

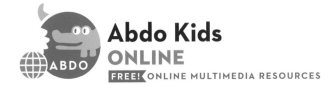

24